3&5 SUPER SECRET METHOD TO ENLARGE YOUR PENIS SIZE

USING NATURAL & HERBAL METHOD

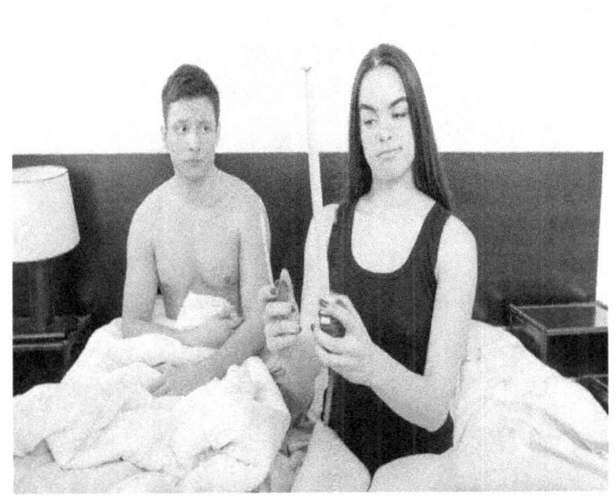

TABLE OF CONTENTS

SECTION A

NATURAL METHOD OF INCREASING YOUR PENIS......13
PENIS ENLARGEMENT EXERCISES MYTH OR FACT
HOW BIG CAN YOU GET?
Fundamental tips to get you started
SMART MOVES TO MAKE IT LOOK BIGGER
INTRODUCING THE PC MUSCLE OR PC FLEX
ENDING YOUR WORKOUT
WORKOUT CONCLUSION

SECTION B

HOW TO INCREASE PENIS SIZE USING HERBS
PART 1: Using Herbs to Increase Blood Flow to the Penis
PART 2: EXTRA TIPS
PART 3: KNOWING WHAT TO AVOID

DISCLAIMER

DEDICATION

This book is Dedicated to all men of Good Will – who with their support this book is published and also to all that bring out their time to read this wonderful life changing book.

ACKNOLOWLEDGEMENT

Special Thanks to all my esteemed readers around the world. God bless you for your patronage. You are my strength. I appreciate even as you give me good recommendation. I will not fail you. I am poised to give you my best. Continue to read and don't give up!

SUPER SECRET METHOD TO ENLARGE YOUR PENIS SIZE

SECTION A: 3 Super Ancient And Modern Secrets That Will Explode Your Penis Size, Man Power, Turn Your Sexual Confidence 360^0 And Make You A Sex Machine In Less Than Few Weeks.

SECTION B: 5 Super Herbal Substance/Medicine That Will Unleash Your Penis Size, Man Power, Turn Your Sexual Confidence 360^0 And Make You A Sex Machine In Less Than Few Weeks.

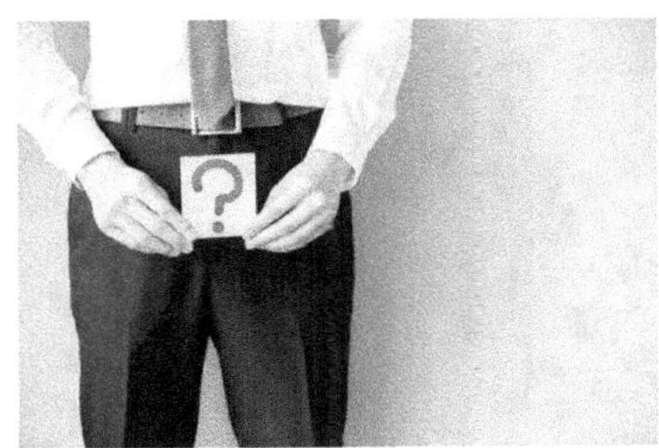

In this special report, you are going to learn ultimate secrets to __naturally gain more penis length/girth and how to last longer during sex, giving you ultimate control__.

But First, Why did I create this report?

I want you to take a look at these pictures

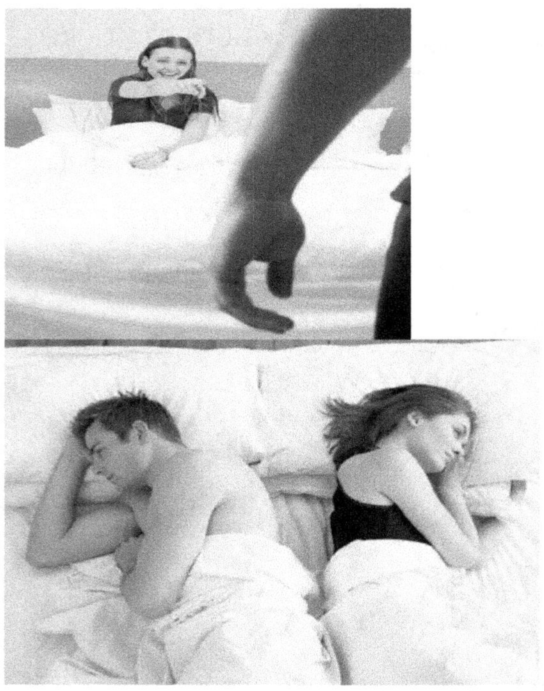

In the first picture; you can see that the woman was laughing at the man's arsenal because of the small size.

Are you having such experience or something close?

In the second picture; the once in love couple are finally getting a divorce because of the man's inability to satisfy the wife sexually.

Are you having such experience or something close?

Do you want to never experience the above?

Then I created this guide for you.

INTRODUCTION

The question most men probably ask upon hearing about natural penis enlargement exercises or learning about this guide for the first time is...hey man! Can this be possible?

Ok come to think of it, the man who goes to the gym constantly to train his muscles to become bigger, stronger and more athletic gets to have his desired goal if he trains right and eats right, don't they? And you get to see that young slim man become a six pack, macho looking athletic bodied man with time, correct?

How about a balloon before you blow it up? You probably stretch it to make the rubber more elastic this enables the balloon hold more air.

Considering these analogies, right, the penis is not a balloon but this procedure also applies with the penis. If the penis is appropriately exercised it can be trained to hold more blood than it does before. It will become surprisingly bigger and lager in size, this includes the girth and length. Amazing right?

Penis enlargement, or **male enhancement**, is any technique aimed to increase the size of a human penis. Some methods aim to increase total length, others the shaft's girth, and yet others the glans size. Techniques include surgery, supplements, ointments, **EXERCISES,** patches, and physical methods like pumping, jelqing, and traction etc.

Listen; there have been a lot of scams all over the world when it comes to what really enhances the size of the penis.

There are millions of products offline and online ranging from pills, pumps, creams etc that are being sold and people are still falling victim to purchasing these products that 90% of them do not work.

Why?

The reason is because a lot of men grow up to find out that while they look handsome on the outside and possess every other feature, they are on the smaller side underneath.

Feels bad right? I know, because I've been there.

There is a whole new world of satisfaction plus benefits to be enjoyed when you have a bigger penis, the confidence it can bring can literally blow your mind, can you remember the last time you wanted to approach a fine woman but didn't have enough confidence to? Or even the last time you went to the gents but felt insecure whilst standing at the urinals? Well that's about to stop,

Amazingly a bigger penis can bring you the confidence to approach that woman you had an interest in with confidence knowing that you can satisfy any woman beyond avalanche, or walk into the gents and feel good using the urinals because you know that you probably might be bigger downstairs than the other folks, this self-confidence can radiate throughout your entire life. Don't believe me? Then continue reading this guide.

This guide was created from wealth of knowledge gotten from experiences, best practices and scientific backings concerning penis health and natural hands on exercises that has being thoroughly packaged to help you

- Enlarge you penis to your desired size
- Measure it appropriately
- Control the addition in size
- Control Erect le dysfunction

I am sure, because I have tried some of them with great success, and I have received tons of positive reviews from around the world from men who got this guide from me and used it.

REASONS FOR SEEKING PENIS ENLARGEMENT

Some men seeking penis enlargement have normal-sized penises, and many may experience *penile dysmorphophobia* by underestimating their own penis size while overestimating the average penis size. Other men may want a larger penis to enhance their sex lives, even if their penis is average or above average in size already. Couples might want one or both partners to enlarge their penis size if they have a fetish for large penises. A larger penis may also play into BDSM and S&M, with a dominant male intentionally having a large penis to inflict pain upon their partner during sexual intercourse.

SECTION A

NATURAL METHOD OF INCREASING YOUR PENIS SIZE

PENIS ENLARGEMENT EXERCISES MYTH OR FACT

Many men horridly disbelieve penis exercises as sweet talks or myths without trying to find out in depth on its facts. Penis exercises have been practised in different forms from generations. Primitively, usage of weights, different objects and workouts has enhanced the structure of different body parts, to achieve new looks.

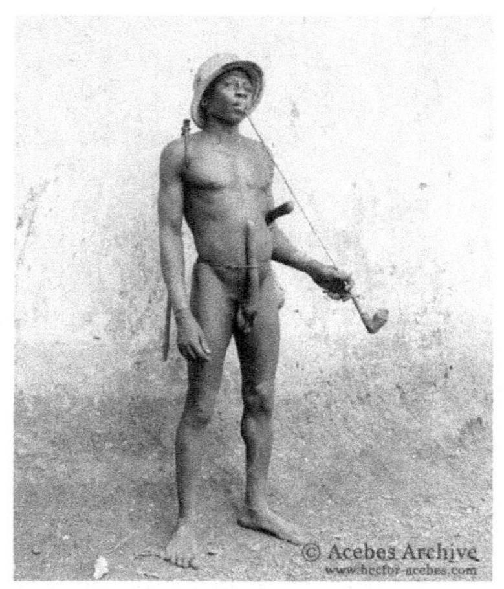

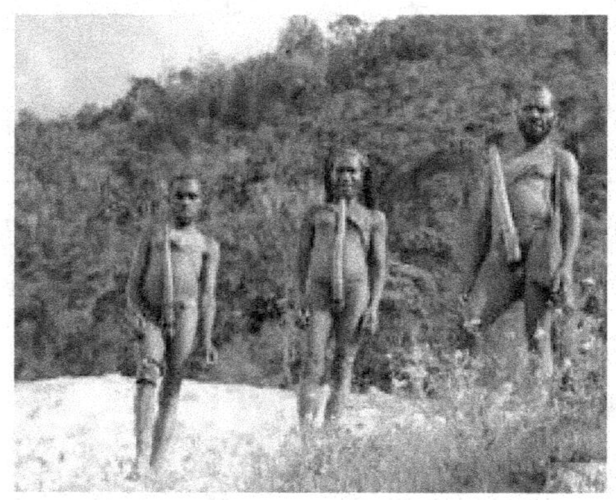

This native African who is about to be initiated into manhood put his penis in it for some months until it reaches a particular desired size and length then he removes it.

Surely it was found early enough that the human body can be improved consciously using devices or exercises. The ancient men used weights or carved wood with hole where the penis is inserted and tied (see above image) for a long period of time as tool to gain penis enlargement.

The concept behind body enhancement is the adaptability of the human body as response to external stimuli. Just as the extra physical effort put into working out at the gym will trigger an increase in size of the muscles that have sustained the effort.

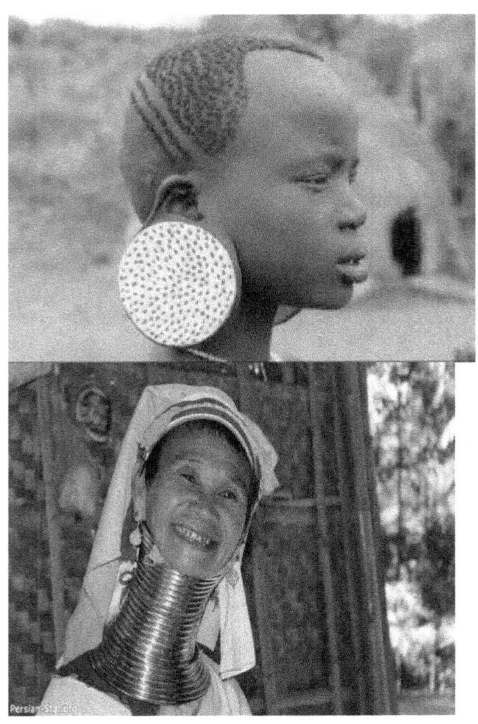

Similarly constant exercises on the penis will cause the body to start multiplying the cells that makes up the penis tissues and force it to accept more blood which results to increase in both length and girth of the penis.

HOW BIG CAN YOU GET?

Take a good look at the chart below first to have an idea of what your goals should look like.

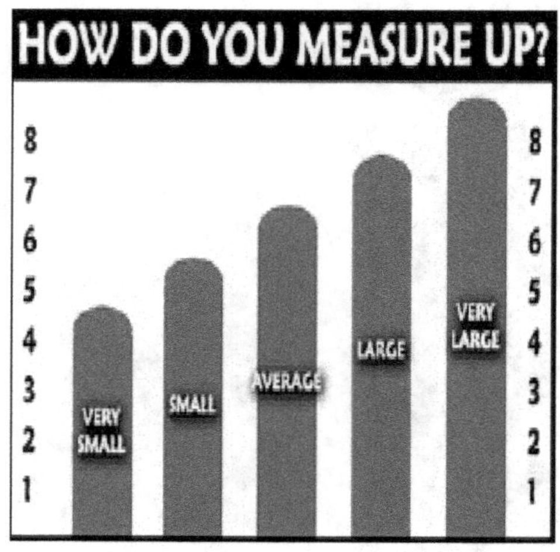

Ideally, I don't think any man needs a penis that is above 7 inches but it is left for you to decide based on your immediate size and your goal.

The penis looks simple and so precise that both males and females think they know all about it.

But the penis is a complex organ that is made up of two parts: the shaft and the glens (the head). The shaft is not a muscle as some think. It is made of three columns of tissue which are called the corpus spongiosus, which forms the underside of the penis and the glens and the corpora cavernosa, which are two chambers of tissue

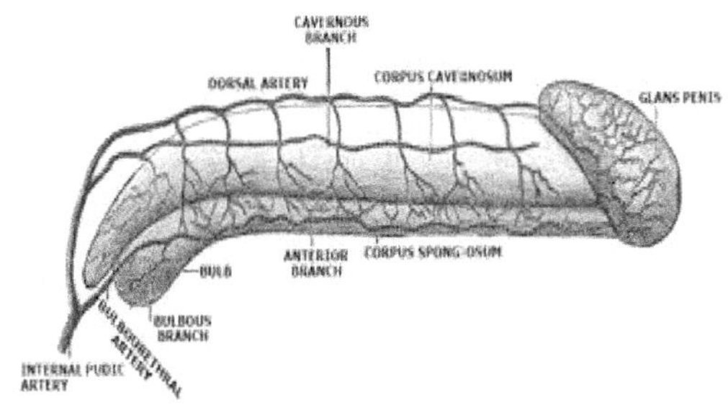

Located next to eachother on the upperside

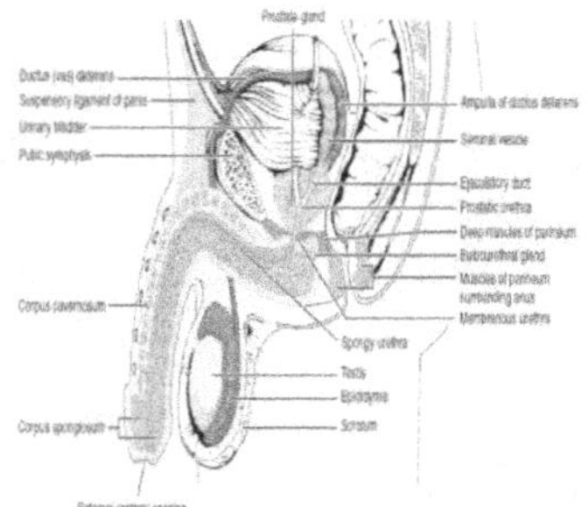

of the penis.

Erection can be achieved by filling the two corpora cavernosa chambers with blood, unlike some animals, humans poses no erectile bone and has to depend on engorgement with blood to achieve erection.

If you can perform these workouts right, these chambers will eventually be able to hold more blood. This leads to a lager penis.

Note: growing the penis means expanding the erectile tissue.

After engaging in your first penis enlargement exercise in some weeks you'll gain 1.5 inches rapidly in your flaccid size. At same stage you'll gain about 1 inch in erect size.

For instance, if you are currently 7.5 inches, your penis will probably not grow 3 inches to 10.5. If your erect penis is currently 5.0 inches, then expect that it will be around 6.5 inches within about 90 days.

Note: Penis growth rate depends largely on how fast your body adapts to expansive growth. There are majorly 4 types of penis size gainers.

KINDS OF PENIS SIZE GAINERS

1. There are men who are able to easily increase both in girth and length fast.
2. There are men who can easily increase the length of their penis.
3. There are men who easily increase in girth of their penis
4. Finally there are men who are slow to increasing both length and girth of their penis.

Which these groups do you belong?

Well you cannot know until you start.

Make sure you read this guide thoroughly and choose which exercises are best for you.

There are amazingly effective techniques in this guide, stick to them and watch your little man grow bigger.

<u>Here are fundamental tips to get you started.</u>

The first thing you should keep in mind when starting penis enlargement program is that you really need to put your willpower behind this. Just like everything else achievable you need to stick to penis enlargement to see results.

Don't start something just to find out two weeks later that it bores the hell out of you. Penis **enlargement works** only if you strive to do the exercises right and stick to a regular routine.

MAKE SURE YOU MEASURE YOUR PENIS FIRST

FLACCID: Get a ruler or a measuring tape and place it over your penis. Then push the ruler back into your abdomen as far as it will go. Hold your limp (flaccid) penis along the ruler and measure to the tip of the head.

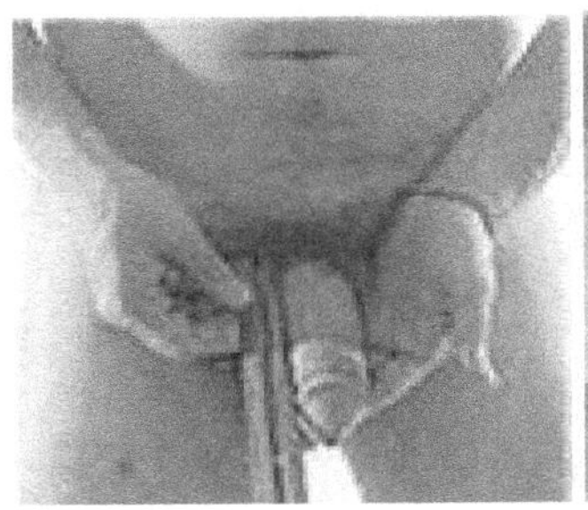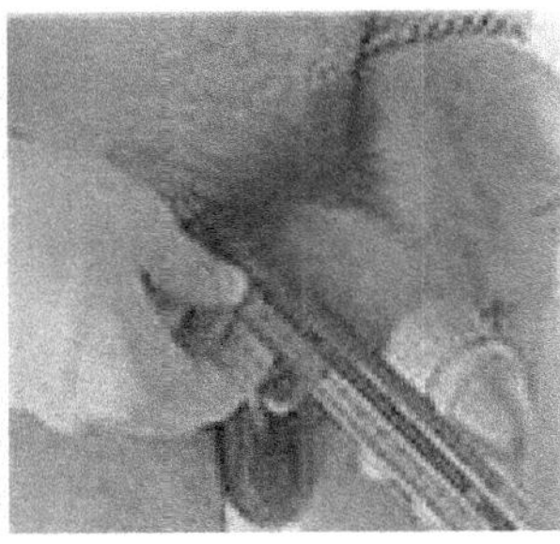

Note: The length of the flaccid penis can be dictated by many things, including the temperature. This means contradicting results depending on the temperature or the situation that you are in. Flaccid gains are often the first gains you will notice when performing penis enlargement exercises.

ERECT: While standing, gently angle your erect penis until its parallel to the floor. Press the ruler against your pubic bone (just above the base of the penis) then measure from top to tip.

It may be easier to measure by standing with your knees locked and grabbing the penis from the bottom, just behind the head on either side.

Press the ruler against your pubic bone, and measure on top of penis as you pull it out as far as you can. Try moving your pelvis or changing the angle to see what variations can occur during this type of measurement.

Once you've figured out how to measure to get the same result as your erect length, you will find that this measurement is easier and more convenient when measuring your actual size.

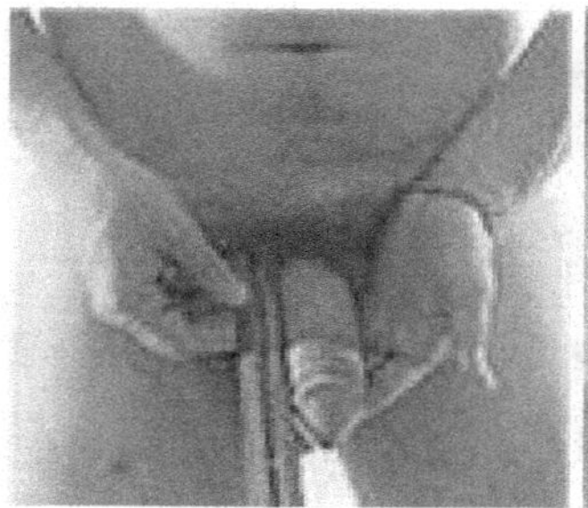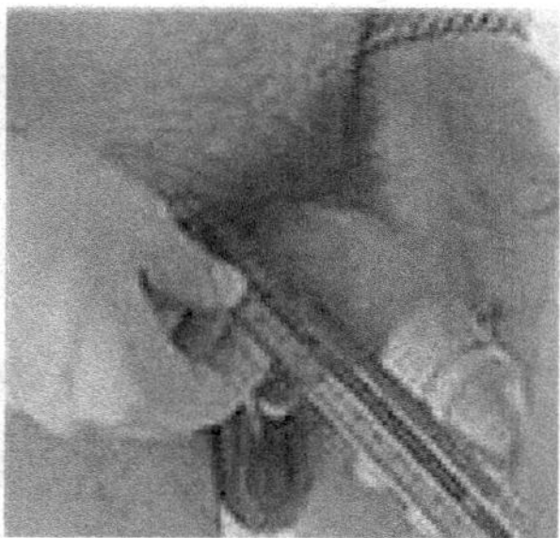

THICKNESS/GIRTH: The girth can be extremely awkward to measure because many people have different size girth measurements depending on which part of the penis that you measure. The standard way is to measure in the centre of the penis shaft.

When flaccid hold your penis out in front of you and wrap a tape measure around your penis. Do not pull the tape measure too hard. Pull it to a reasorable level and remember this amount of pull next time you measure. The average flaccid girth size is between 3"-4; In the photographs the model has a large flaccid length and girth and it is likely that yours will be smaller.

With a piece of cloth measuring tape, measure the circumference of your erect penis at the mid-penis shaft.

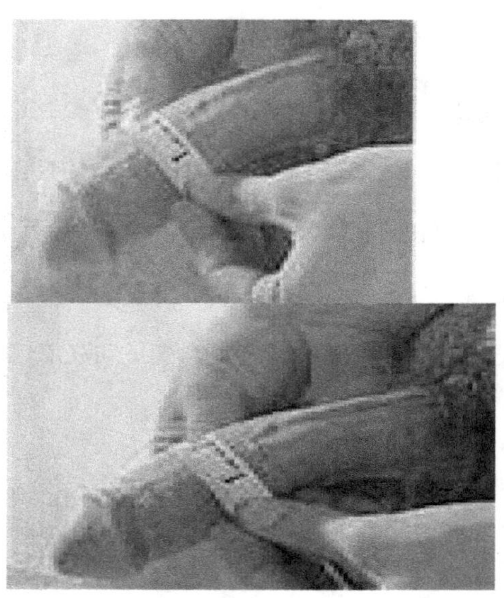

Measuring the Erect Girth: make sure your penis is 100% erect and then proceed with the measuring tape. Hold your penis in front of you so it's parallel with the floor. With your other hand place the tape measure around the penis making sure not to pull too tight. The average erect girth is 5′5′-′6′according to recent surveys, but more is always better and more admirable.

Measure around the penis and make a note of your measurement.

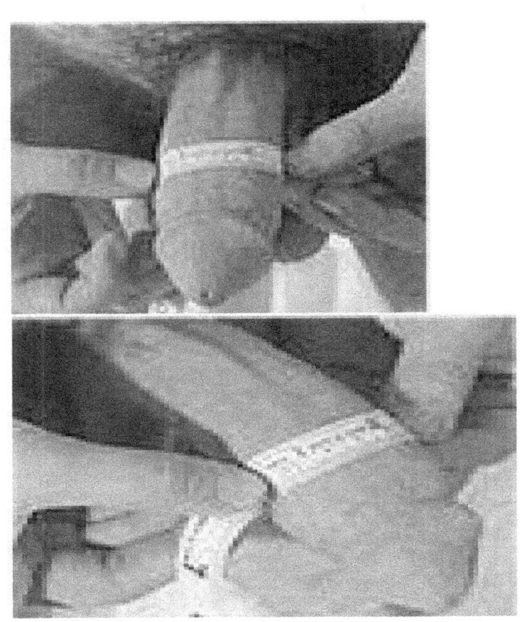

Tracking Your Gains:

Yes; the reason you are embarking on a penis enlargement program is to **increase the size of your manhood**, thereby increasing the value. Therefore it makes sense to keep track on your gains. You can use a table like the one shown below to record your starting measurements and then update them every 4-6 weeks. By keeping track you will help to keep yourself motivated when you start to see the gains you were hoping for!

	Start	Date and Measurement								
Flaccid Length										
Erect Length										
Flaccid Girth										
Erect Girth										

Don't exaggerate! This is something you aren't going to show to anybody else (unless you want to) and there's no reason to lie to yourself.

If you exaggerate now, you won't be able to correctly identify gains in the future, which usually leads to demonization and failure. Don't measure yourself too often, once every four or six weeks is enough to show you how much you've gained.

Don't expect results to appear overnight. It may take a month or more for the first gains to show up. Just stay in the course and you'll **reach your goal**. The penis is tissue and not muscle, so whereas muscle are fast to grow in size as response to a genuine need, the penis is simply tissue and it takes much longer to force tissue to expand.

If you're interested in **good results and safe enlargement,** you could join a professional program of penis enlargement exercises. The best programs come with **detailed explanation, photos and videos** in order to make sure that you perform the exercises correctly every time and will offer you a dedicated support team should you have questions that need answering.

You can also follow up on our upcoming guides, videos, Images and penis tips that will be emailed to our subscribers.

Penis enlargement routines are usually preceded and followed by warm up and down sessions. It's important that you do not skip these sessions. They help get your penis ready for a good workout and for the healing and rebuilding process that follows exercises. Warm up sessions decreases the risk of injuries, while warming down helps the penis to heal faster.

Remember that there are no set routines. Feel free to experiment with the exercises and find out what works for you.

SMART MOVES TO MAKE IT LOOK BIGGER

<u>Tips to encourage your process</u>.

CUT YOUR PUBIC HAIR:_Not only does this make your penis look bigger, but it helps when you're doing some of these exercises. You can just give it a **low cut**. When **stretching, pulling, and milking** your penis, you don't want to be pulling your hairs.

LOSE WEIGHT: It is estimated that for every 30 pounds overweight you are, you lose one inch in length because of its hidden underneath your fat.

EAT HEALTHY AND TAKE VITAMINS: In order to eliminate any possibility of slow growth, make sure you're getting ample amount of nutrients. This works like when a body builder is trying to develop bigger and stronger muscles.

He has to eat very well and take good vitamins.

The proper levels of minerals, amino acids, and vitamins **do** have an effect on the workout process.

Also drink lots of water!

PSYCHOLOGIC CONDITIONING: Most importantly, have a good/growth state of mind. Your mentality has a lot to do with the growth of your penis. If you don't believe that this enlargement of a thing will work, it's very likely that your subconscious will make it more difficult to physically grow your penis. A positive attitude is essential.

EXERCISE IT LIKE YOU DO THE REST OF YOUR BODY:

You go to the gym to tone up, get the blood pumping and to make certain muscles bigger. You can do the same with your penis and the following sections will tell you **exactly** what to do.

100% ALL NATURAL EXERCISE

Just as we've said, in order to see real gains, these exercises demand **COMPLETE 100%** devotion.

You must perform them for at least **5 DAYS A WEEK**.

If at any time you begin to feel discomfort or pain, take a little time off. You want to enlarge your penis not hurt it.

Remember, by applying tension, pulling, stretching, or expansion to a penis you are creating a force which will spilt the cells in the penis.

You want to be sure to spilt the cell and break it down just enough to ensure structural balance on a safe level as to allow for the normal healing process (like a body builder would do).

By forcing the division of too many cells, because of too much pressure, you are creating ugly healing which will create a distorted penis, possibly with no rate of gains.

Please..... DO NOT OVER DO IT!!!!!

If performed correctly and routinely, you will soon begin to see the results you hope for.

Within the first few weeks or so, your penis will actually start looking LONGER AND THICKER. That should be all the encouragement you need to keep up with your daily exercises!

When performing the Jelqing exercise (you will get more information about it later), you will need to apply a **lubricant** on your penis.

For the lubricant, Please **Do Not Use Soap or Shampoo!**

As these can irritate the skin when applied so vigorously for so long on the skin. It can also dry out the skin severely, causing it to crack and peel for a few days. More so, it can sting if it gets into the hole (the urethral opening) at the end of your penis.

Vaseline (petroleum jelly) works, but... be forewarned....its greasy and makes a mess. Another downside is that Vaseline is so thick; it may not allow you to move your hand as fast as you'd like.

Baby oil also works, but is also very messy and leaves stains.

One of the best bets is using **Vaseline intensive care.** It cleans up fairly easily, is slippery, it lasts long, and lets you go as fast as you want when performing the exercises.

Be aware of when and when not to engage in penis enlargement.

If you have a disease which may alter blood circulation, oxygenation, and regeneration of tissues like advanced diabetics, respiratory instability, and cirrhosis, consult an urologist.

As you're doing your workout, here are some symptoms to be aware of.

- Blisters are a result of too much pressure on the penis for a prolonged period of time. You want pressure, but don't overdo it.
- Red sores are a result of too much stretch. In order to avoid this, hold off on your exercise until the blisters have disappeared.
- "Fuzzy skin" is a result of tissue abuse. When you touch this affected area you can actually feel its fuzziness because

it's directly external. This is the partially dead tissue covering your penis. This can happen when too much tension is applied. Red sores sometimes accompany fussy skin.

That being said, **the exercises we're about to discuss are all healthy and natural ways to produce penis growth**.

Just use good sense when performing them. We recommend a daily workout which should be performed 5days a week, but if at any time you begin to feel real pain or discomfort, **please ease up**.

Note: YOU SHOULD NOT RUSH THROUGH THESE EXERCISES IN AN ATTEMPT TO SPEED UP THE PROCESS.

DOING MORE THEN YOU CAN HANDLE IS A RECIPE FOR OVERTRAINING.

RECOMMENDED ROUTINES

Below you will find 3 recommended starter routines. The first of which incorporates all of the exercises which we will give you later on this guide. While it is possible to see gains using the shortest routine, you may want to consider signing up to a <u>full exercise program </u>to enable you get access to more advanced exercises to really enhance and speed up your gains.

Basic Beginner Routine

Exercise Name	Minutes	Target Area
The Wake Up Cloth	2	Blood Flow
The Long Schlong	3	Length
The Jelq	3	Length & Girth
Horizontal Movement	2	Girth
The Wake Up Cloth	2	Blood Flow
PC Flex Basic	50 Reps	Girth & Control

Regular Beginner Routine

Exercise Name	Minutes	Target Area
The Wake Up Cloth	3	Blood Flow
The Long Schlong	5	Length
The Jelq	8	Length & Girth
The Power Stretch	4	Length
Horizontal Movement	3	Girth
The Wake Up Cloth	2	Blood Flow
PC Flex Basic	100 Reps	Girth & Control

Extended Beginner Routine

Exercise Name	Minutes	Target Area
The Wake Up Cloth	3	Blood Flow
The Long Schlong	8	Length
The Jelq	10	Length & Girth
The Power Stretch	6	Length
Horizontal Movement	5	Girth
Needling	3	Head Size
The Wake Up Cloth	3	Blood Flow
PC Flex Basic	150 Reps	Girth & Control

WARM UPS FOR THE EXERCISES

The warm-up is **ESSENTIAL.** You should never leave the warm-up out of your routine as this will lead to gains being minimal. It also a good idea to finish off a workout with a "warm down" which would be, for example, the procedure below repeated. A thorough warm up not only helps with the effectiveness of your exercises but also helps prevent against injury by promoting greater blood flow.

To perform this warm up you will need a cloth or small/hand towel and access to warm water. Firstly find an ample sized face cloth. Wet it with warm water until it is soaked and hot but still manageable. Then wrap the cloth around your penis (either flaccid or erect) hold it there for a minute. When 1 minute is up, repeat it a couple of times increasing the rounds to about 2minutes if comfortable for you. (See below image).

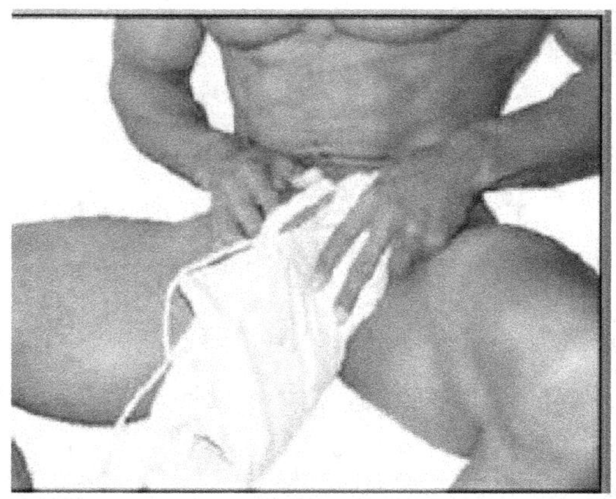

After the warm up, make sure to dry off your penis well before moving on to the next.

Why Hot Water?

Heat makes the penis more flexible, more relaxed and less stiff. The main reason for warming up is so when you're exercising you aren't tearing a stiff tissue within your penis. Instead, you're exercising relaxed flexible tissue and the more flexible your penis, the easier it stretches, and the more it enlarges.

What the hotness does is to draw blood to the area of your penis, increasing the blood flow and making the skin slightly elastic. This also ensures a good grip for the exercises you will perform.

NOTE: Keep the warm up away from your testicles as much as possible. Your testicles do not like heat. So keep the hot towel away from them.

Also make sure that you warm up the perineum; the per neum is the area between your testicles and your anus and that is where your inner penis is located.

The Long Schlong or Stretching Exercise

Please make sure you are thoroughly warmed up and ready. Make sure that your penis is always completely limp and flaccid –it's both difficult and dangerous to perform these exercises if you have full erection.

Take the head of your penis in your hand (if you have a foresk n then pull this back so it does not get in the way, remember you are pulling the penis NOT the skin). Then stretch it out directly in front of you. Holding it about 20-30 seconds.

If you really want to enlarge your penis, this is the technique a lot of men can swear by. You can perform this while standing, lying down or sitting down.

This is stretching and it is indispensable if you want length increase in your penis. You will have to do about 3-5 minutes of stretching per day.

The goal of stretching it slowly gets your penis used to the stretch.

Step 1: with your penis in its flaccid state, take one hand and grip it firmly. Anywhere will do as long as it is not directly on the penis cap. Be careful not to cut off too much circulation.

See image below:

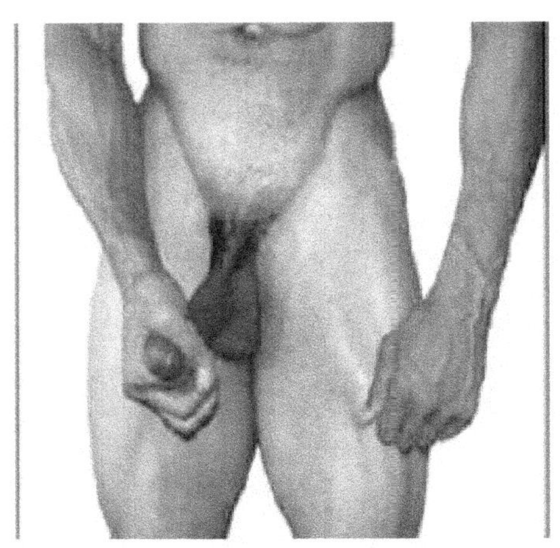

Step 2: Pull your penis out directly in front of yourself. Stretch it as much as you can without causing pain or discomfort. Hold it there for about 30 seconds. After each round, pull it out slightly further each time.

Step 3: Relax for one minute. "Twirl" your penis in a circular motion about 30 times. This gets circulation flowing again.

Step 4: Repeat step two again four times, except pull your penis in a different position each time (right, left, up and down). After each 30 seconds pull. Repeat step 3.

Step 5: After you've completed 5 pulls (30 seconds each), pull your penis out directly in front of you one more time. Give it a good 1-minute stretch and 10 slight "tugs" outward, not jerking too hard.

Stretching the penis with your hand produces the same results as traditional penis weight systems.

There is nothing wrong designing your peculiar way of gripping your penis, as long as you know where and where not to apply the wrong pressures. Again, DON'T HOLD TOO TIGHT, otherwise you'll cut off the circulation.

This exercise will ensure a longer penis within 2 weeks, but within 3-4 months it will really be noticeable.

Common Question: Can I hold each stretch longer than 30 seconds?

Answer: It is advisable that you use the 30 seconds basic when you're just start out.

Over the next 5 weeks, you can increase it up to 60 seconds per stretch.

STRETCHING TECHNIQUE TWO

This technique is very similar to the one a lot of upcoming porn-stars who want to quickly add up 2 inches to their penis, use, and have admitted to using it. It is also known as the JAI stretch.

<u>Here's the instructions:</u>

1. While in its flaccid (limp) state, take one hand and grip around the head of your penis. Grip firmly, but not hard enough to feel discomfort 0r cut off too much circulation. (<u>Remember</u>; pull gently)
2. Pull out directly in front of yourself with enough force to feel a good and painless stretch in your penis. Hold and

count for at least 30 seconds to one minute and....

3. Release the stretch for about 2 seconds before you stretch again.

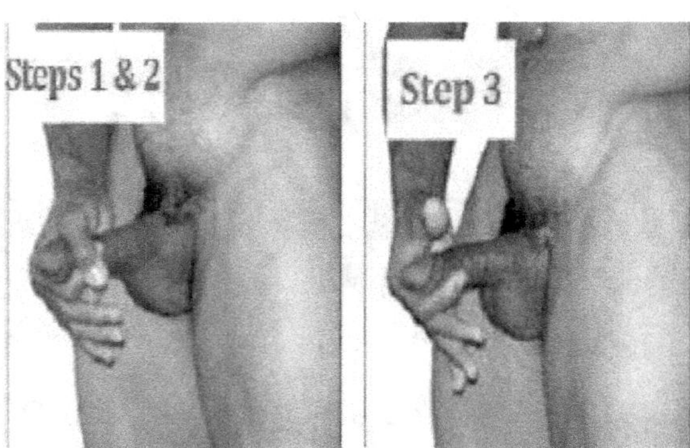

Then continue until you've logged in 5-20 minutes of session.

STRETCHING TECHNIQUE THREE

This version of stretching appears in a bestselling book on male sexuality. It also involves stretching the penis in both its flaccid and erect state.

1. With your right hand grip the penis and rhythmically pull it forward and away from your body 10 times (roughly 15 seconds each pull).
2. Repeat to the right (10 times) to force energy into the head.
3. Rub the head of your penis with your thumb and forefinger. Pull forward an inch (10 times) to force energy into head.
4. Pull the erect penis to the right and rotate in small circle while pulling outward (10 times). Repeat to the left (10times) and do the same.
5. Gently slap your erect penis against your inner thigh while putting out on each side (10 times).

Those are the stretching techniques. You basically need to choose 1 or 2 of them to use in your routine.

Next....let's talk about a different form of enlargement that not only helps you to add length but it also helps for increasing your girth and hardness.

It's known as Jelqing.

THE JELQING EXERCISE

Often dubbed an 'exercise,' jelquing is a technique for penis enlargement that's become popular with the rise of the internet as how-to videos, and online blogs have pushed it as an easy way to make your penis larger. Jelquing refers to penis massage with a hand-over-hand motion to push blood from the base of the penis to the head.

While there are many anecdotal reports online that jelquing is an effective way to increase penis size, no scientific studies have ever concluded that the technique works. Proponents of jelquing claim that regularly stretching and pulling the penis will make the tissue fill with blood, causing it to permanently swell. However, basic penis anatomy contradicts this idea, since the penis is an organ and not a muscle that you can alter or strengthen with penis enlargement exercise. There's also the risk of penile damage with jelquing, since this technique may lead to irritation, blood vessel tears, scar formation, bruising, pain, and desensitization of the penis.

This exercise is one of the core penis enlargement exercises. The jelq supposedly originated in the Arabic culture. The story goes that a large penis was seen as a mark of power and Arabians did this exercise to enlarge their penis. Whether this is true or not is irrelevant, the fact is this exercise works.

The main function of the jelq is to strengthen and thicken the penis. It works by filling the Corpora Cavernosa with more blood than normal. The excess blood allows the area to be stretched further and further. The workout breaks down fibre, which grow back bigger than before.

Over the course of several months, the blood spaces in the penis become larger, which means that they can hold more blood. This in return makes your penis larger and also helps you get harder erections.

We have found that there are **several** different variations of jelqing that are practiced by men. The general notion of "milking the penis" is always the same, but the techniques seem to vary a bit.

Our personal preference is TECHNIQUE ONE. We have more success growth-wise with our clients with this particular technique. Read through all different variations on jelqing and decide which technique you think would for you.

You will want use a lubricant tor these exercises.

The results from jelqing are PERMANENT. The penis will become enlarged in both the flaccid and erect state.

The exercises are beneficial, not harmful. They will actually **improve the health and strength** of the male organ as well as **increase its size.**

Jelqing doesn't require extreme pressure for work it to work. The goal is to push the blood up the penis, not force it. Use a graceful, light grip.

IMPORTANT: Care must be taken that the exercise is NOT PERFORMED DURING HARD ERECTION.

Vascular (vein) damage could result if the penis is forcibly milked in its fully erect state. You want your penis to be between half ¾ erect.

Results cannot be obtained until a partial erection is present. After this exercise has been performed, it will be noticed that the penis (even in its flaccid state) appears both longer and thicker. That is a fact.

And from within one to several months of exercise, the penis will appear rather enormous; this is due to the impaction of blood in the penile tissues.

Choose ONE of the jelqing exercise techniques below to include in your workout.

This simple exercise, if practiced five days a week, will enable a man who possesses, for example, a six-inch erect penis, to add from between one to three inches to the length of his penis <u>(measured at the top, from tip to pelvis)</u> and it will grow in circumference proportionately.

Little or no growth may be apparent for approximately one month. During the second or third month an increase of two or more inches will be common.

Remember to warm up for about ten minutes before attempting to jelq.

JELQING TECHNIQUE ONE

1-When your penis is **<u>semi-erect;</u>** use your thumb and forefinger to form a circle like in the picture below. With this hand, grip tightly around the base of your penis (as close to your pubic bone as possible. (Note; your penis must be lubr cated at this stage).

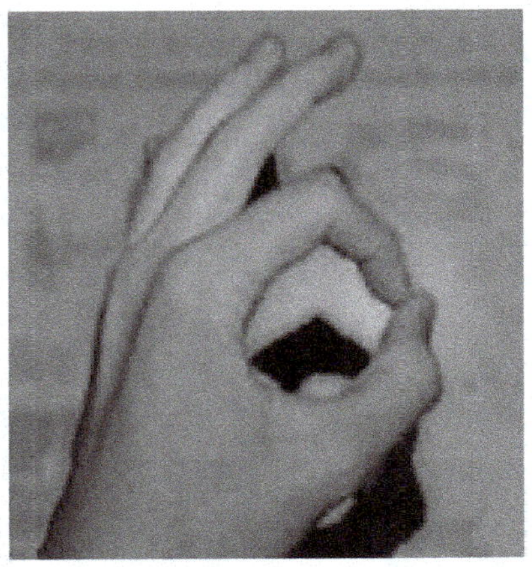

2- Now starting from the base, pull the penis gently but firmly, stretch downward and outward.

Your penis should still be in a semi-erect state. Make sure to touch the penis all the way from the base to the head. Stop the grip directly before you reach the head (cup) of the penis. Each jelq should take about 3 seconds.

See Image Below:

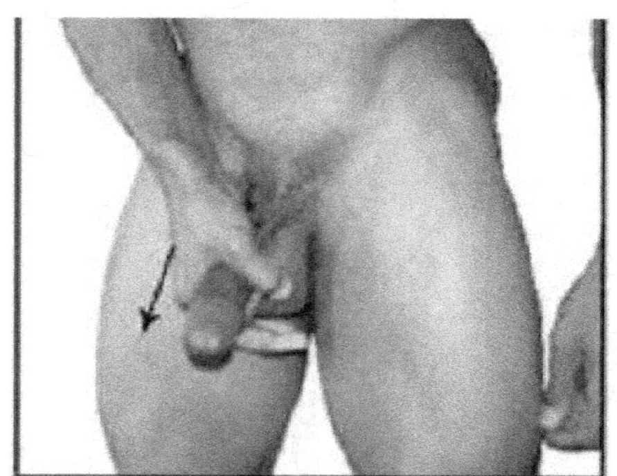

3- Switch to the second hand and do the same thing. Start from the base and stretching downward to the head. Alternate both hands in a smooth rhythmic ("milking") motion, touching upon every part of the penis except the very top part of the penis head.

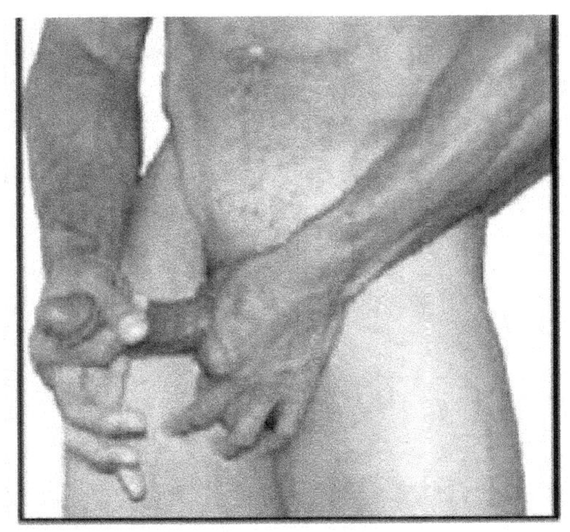

Do 200-300 strokes/day at medium strength for the first 2 weeks. (10 minutes)

Do 300-500mstrokes/day at medium-full strength for the next week. (15 minutes)

If you find yourself getting an erection during this exercise, squeeze harder to discourage it or s mply wait until it subsides. You can encourage circulation afterward by slapping your penis up and down 25-50 times. Perform this exercise 5 days a week.

Remember to keep your penis only partially erect. If you feel ejaculation coming on, pause milking until the urge subsides. This itself is an exercise...one of self-control that will help you last longer when having sex.

JELQING TECHNIQUE TWO

1- Apply Lubrication to the flaccid penis from the handle of the penis to the head.

2- Using only the thumb and forefinger, stretch the penis downward and slightly outward. Be gentle, but firm.

3- Alternate hands, one then the other, in a "milking action".

4- keep performing gently until a certain amount of swelling develops, then perform the action a **bit** firmly and forcibly.

5- Repeat this action 100 times.

For the ten days, rake it relatively easy. Gradually though, you should be performing 200 repetitions. These exercises are same for both circumcised and uncircumcised men. It will be noticed that the head (or glans) will swell considerably. This s normal and good, and is due to the forcing of blood to that area.

JELQING TECHNIQUE THREE

This is the "DRY" version of jelqing and you can use this in nstances when you are outside using a public toilet.

It is just as if you are doing either Techniques 1 or 2, but without the lubricant.

IN "dry" milking you squeeze and pull the skin, but you don't slide your fingers over the skin. As the penis becomes too large to cover in one stroke, work on the base and middle of the shaft separately.

Some guys like to milk "dry" in the morning before getting out of bed (when testosterone levels are the highest). If you find our penis is getting sore, take a day off.

JELQUING TECHNIQUE FOUR

This is also known as Tao technique.

This works for men who want a bigger "mushroom" head on their penis. It's essentially the same as Technique One, except performed slower and more gently.

Use your fingers to push the blood up to your penis head and create some sustained pressure. Hold that position momentarily (approximately 10 seconds).

This will expand the capacity of your head to take in more blood, in the end creating a bell or mushroom shape. You can also squeeze she shaft to make the blood engorge in the head.

Once it's hard, you can release the squeeze. Repeat as many times as you wish (but don't exceed 10 mins).

That is all about the main exercises.

INTRODUCING THE PC MUSCLE OR PC FLEX

There are penis exercises that involve what is called the PC MUSCLE.

The PC muscle is what can help you to last for as long as you want in bed.

Performing these PC muscle exercises are important for several reasons:

- They give you stronger erections.
- They create intense (sometimes multiple) orgasms.
- They help you to control your ejaculation.
- They help you to shorten the recovery time between orgasms.
- They help you to develop a healthy prostrate.

The PC muscle or (pubococcygeal muscle) is actually a group of pelvic muscles that form the basis of your sexual health.

They run from your pubic bone in the front to your tailbone in the back. You can feel this muscle at your perineum, just behind your testicles and in front of your anus.

In simple terms, this is the muscle that you can use to stop urine when you are urinating. The next time you are urinating, try to stop the flow of urine several times. The muscle that makes that happen is the PC muscle.

For men, this is the muscle that involuntarily "pumps" when you ejaculate.

Strengthening and learning to control this muscle, you will find, is what I call; **The Ultimate Sex Secret that Most Men Never Discover and Use.**

These PC exercises involve doing a set of easy-to-learn pelvic-muscle exercises.

This is a FOOLPROOF way for men to boost their partners' and their own pleasure during lovemaking. Women have already been using their PC muscles for years to help them get sexually aroused easier, lubricate faster, and have more and better orgasms.

First you must locate your PC muscle.

It's actually easier for men to locate this muscle and do these exercises than it is for women. Simply stop your urine midstream when you urinate. This not only teaches you how to find the PC muscle, but gets you started on your exercises.

Stop and restart your urination 5 times during every trip to the bathroom. Using your ability to stop the flow of urine will help you control your ejaculations.

Ancient techniques refer to this process simply as "tightening the anus" because that is what you are indirectly doing when flexing the PC muscles. You can flex the PC muscle quickly and repeatedly, or clench tight and hold for as long as you can.

This latter exercise is tougher than it sounds, yet this is the exercise that will help you prolong your erections and increase the force with which you ejaculate.

Once you've found your PC muscle, you can start doing the PC Exercises anytime, anywhere. You want to squeeze your PC a daily basis.

THESE ARE THE PC EXERCISES:

1. **Perform quick PC CLAMPS:** *Squeeze and release, over and over, start with sets of twenty, and then build to 100 or more. Do at least 250 PC clamps every day, for the rest of your sexual active life.*

Your goal is to be capable of creating 1,000 clamps a day.

Practise LONG SQUEEZES by holding the PC muscle clamped tightly for thirty seconds, or as long as you can.

The way to do the PC clamp is by doing the same thing you do when you want to stop urine.

   2. <u>Try doing STAIR STEPS</u>: *Tighten and loosens in increments. Tighten for a couple of seconds, loosen for a couple of seconds. Do it over and over again.*

   3. <u>PC FLUTTER:</u> *Tighten the PC muscle as slowly as you possibly can. Once you've finished the slow squeeze (to where you can't squeeze anymore), let go. At some point it will "flutter", and you'll feel energy sparkling up your spine. Concentrate on deep, slow breathing while you do this. This is great for restoring energy when you're firing down!*

When you urinate and you want to let those last squirts shoot out, you use your PC muscle in the other direction. By doing this you'll feel your anus open and the sensation is different. This is called the PUSH OUT PC.

Most men can do these exercises anywhere, since they're seldom aroused by the exercises.

Continued over a <u>long period of time,</u> the exercise can help men to get greater arousal, enhanced orgasms and longer-lasting sex. Make these some of the simplest, most beneficial exercises you should do.

EXTRA EXERCISE-DICKS UP

These exercises will strengthen your PC muscle, help improve the blood flow to your penis, and will aid in ejaculatory control.

You can only do this with your penis in an (partially) erect mode.

INSTRUCTIONS:

Flex your PC muscle so that your penis moves up with each flex. Hold it up for about one second with each flex and then drop it down as you relax.

Do this 20 times.

As you get stronger with this, you can increase the length of time for each flex. Like you can lift your penis up and hold it for about 2-3 seconds each.

ADVANCED VERSION: Do this with your towel hanging on the end of your penis. Do 50 repetitions of this and hold each flex for about 5 seconds each.

TIP: You can move to wet towel later on to make it heavier.

See illustrations below:

STEP 1: Hang a small towel over your penis. It may be dry or wet depending on the weight you can carry.

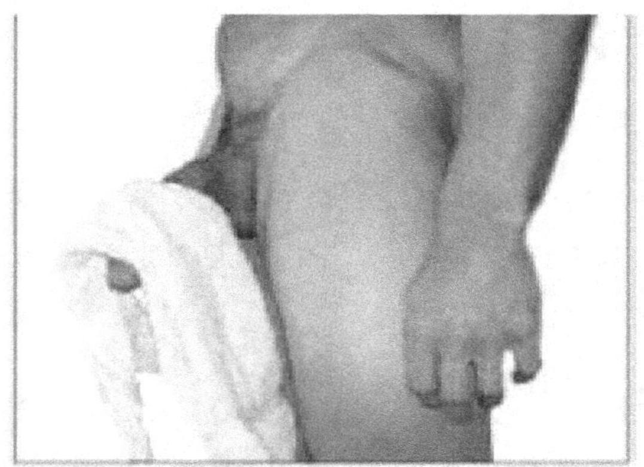

Step 2: Use the erect penis to raise the penis, then lower it, then raise it up again.

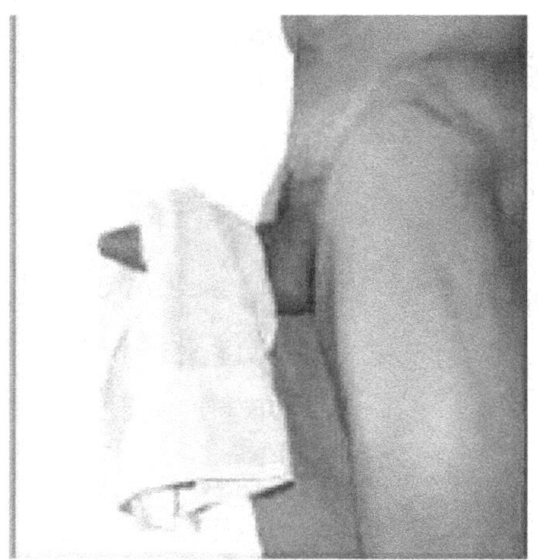

ENDING YOUR WORKOUT

Massage & warm-down

This is how you should end your workout, as applying heat and massage optimizes healing. Your testicles are always trying to maintain a certain temperature to keep the cells alive. So, remember to keep heat away from your testicles. Heat restores any nerve and sensitivity problems you may have incurred during your enlargement program.

After your workout, gently massage your penis for several minutes.

After massage, you can either apply another hot towel as you d d at the beginning of your workout, or you can place your penis in a bowel of lukewarm water for another few minutes.

Either of these "heat application" will keep the blood held within your penis and stimulate the damaged parts, restarting them to function better. Dry off well with a towel.

WORKOUT CONCLUSION

Now that we've explained each of the exercises, it's time to apply them in a daily workout program.

This, my fellow man, is the moment of truth!

If you really want a LARGER PENIS, you must perform these exercises as explained.

These are VERY POWERFUL methods that have been PROVEN!

They're worked for a lot of guys that I know including myself, and they've worked for hundreds of thousands of men throughout history!

So believe me when I say. THEY WILL WORK FOR YOU!!!

This is MY suggested Workout Program.

You MUST do this program for 30 MINUTES DAILY, 5 DAYS A WEEK. Be SURE to take 2days off a week (consecutively or not), as this is your "healing" time when your cells rebuild after they've been broken down.

Do this, and you should start seeing results within the next 3 weeks.

Once you witness this penis growth for yourself, you won't want to stop this program!

REMEMBER...Knowledge, Commitment, and Growth. These exercises have been designed not only for penis enlargement, but also for a better self-esteem and personal satisfaction.

NOTE: For this workout, I have included all recommended techniques for the exercises and you have just read about them.

Whichever technique you decide to use, make sure you stick with them and give them a chance to work. If after a month you find that one of the exercises isn't working for you (which is rarely!), then try a different technique. Always refer to the instruction for ANY of the exercises whenever you need to.

SECTION B:

HOW TO INCREASE PENIS SIZE USING HERBS

If you want to increase the size of your penis, there are several herbs you can use that may stimulate blood flow to the area and temporarily help it get fully erect. More permanent natural solutions to increase its length and width include making dietary changes, getting more exercise and losing weight around your midsection. Much simpler and safer than surgical enhancement, right? See Step 1 to learn more about how you can make your penis larger without resorting to drugs or surgery.

PART 1

Using Herbs To Increase Blood Flow To The Penis

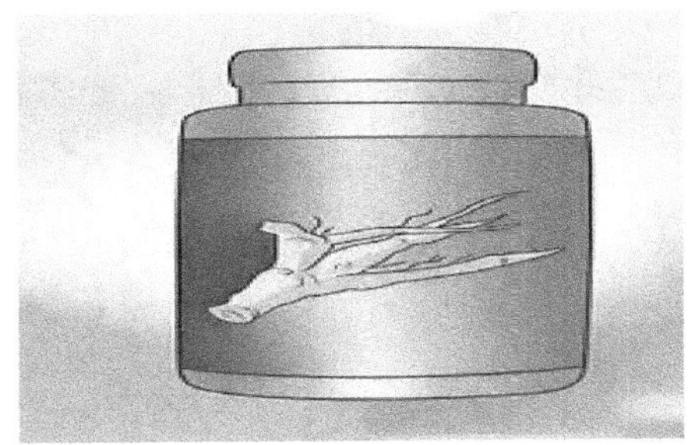

Try ginseng. Korean red ginseng is said to give the nervous system a boost through ginsenosides, a natural component of the plant. While there is no conclusive scientific evidence that ginseng causes the penis to get bigger, men who took ginseng extract tablets as part of a study in South Korea experienced better sexual function after taking the supplements for several weeks.

- Ginseng contraindicates with several medications, and it can have negative side effects for people with certain cancers, heart disease, insomnia, and other disorders. Be sure to talk with your doctor before you begin taking ginkgo regularly.

- If you're considering taking ginseng supplements, look for a supplement labeled "Korean ginseng root" and take 500 mg per day.
- Since herbal supplements are not regulated by the FDA, there is always a risk when taking them. Be sure to purchase the supplements from a reputable company, and never take more than the recommended dosage.

Consider ginkgo biloba.

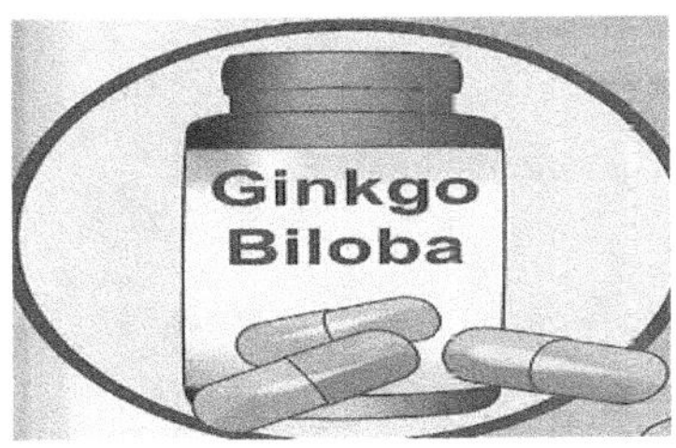

This herb is often taken to boost memory, but it also help with blood circulation and may enhance blood flow to the penis. According to a study conducted at the University of California, ginkgo is most effective at helping men on anti-depressants that can lead to sexual dysfunction. Another study found that gingko had no effect Scientific data is inconclusive, but since gingko enhances memory and has relatively few side effects, it might be worth a try.

- Gingko can be consumed as a tea or a supplement in the form of a capsule. Both forms of the herb are widely available in health food stores.
- Do not take gingko supplements if you have a history of seizures or you're on blood

thinning medication. See your doctor to make sure this supplement is safe for you to take.

Look Into Taking Maca Supplements.

This powder is known for being an aphrodisiac. It contains the photochemicals macamides and macaenes, which are said to boost energy and help men maintain erections. Because no conclusive scientific studies have been conducted on this substance, it's best to proceed with caution. Be sure to discuss it with your doctor before you start adding this supplement to your daily routine.

<u>**Consider taking L-arginine.**</u>

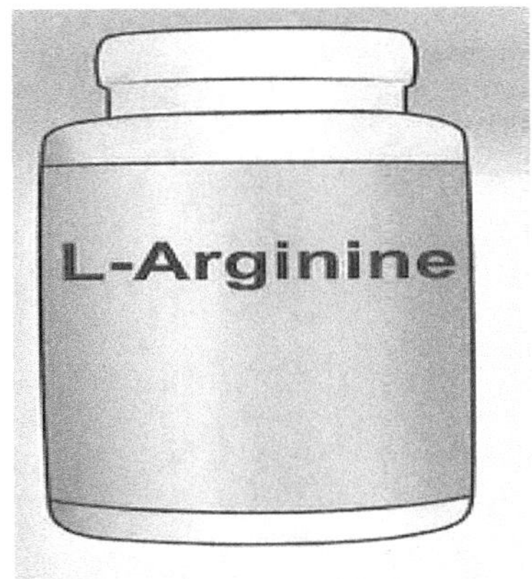

This is an amino acid that leads to increased blood flow, helping the penis get larger during an erection. A study conducted at Tel Aviv University showed that some men experienced improvements after taking the supplement for 6 weeks. It's available in natural food stores, and the recommended dose is 1 gram (0.035 oz) three times a day.[2]

- This supplement should not be taken if you're on nitroglycerin for your heart, because it can cause a drop in blood pressure. Talk with your doctor about whether you should take L-arginine.

<u>Eat watermelon.</u>

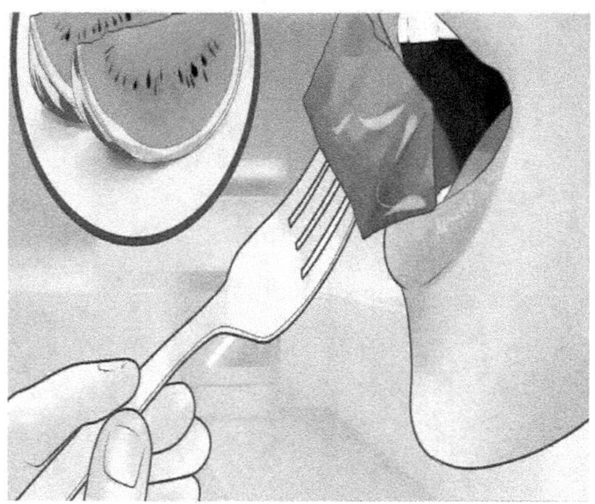

It's not an herb, but it has properties that might help increase the size and duration of erections in a similar way arginine. Watermelon contains an amino acid called citrulline, which gets converted into arginine and leads to the dilation of blood vessels.[4] The fact that watermelon contains citrulline is a relatively new finding, so no studies have been conducted to find out how well it really works or how much watermelon you'd have to eat to see the benefits.

However, since watermelon is considered a superfood when it comes to men's health, you can't go wrong by eating plenty of it while it's in season.

PART 2.

EXTRA TIPS

TRYING SIZE-ENHANCING NATURAL SOLUTIONS

<u>Maintaining a Hard Erection</u>

These tips below will help you achieve longer lasting & harder erections.

Make sure you get plenty of exercises: when you're out of shape, not only does this negatively affect your affect your ability to have sex, it increases the likelihood of erection problems.

I have a set of home workout DVD where I pick one exercise per day and perform it for 30 minutes daily and 4 times in a week.

I call them fat Burning and Libido Boosting workouts.

Watch out for more information about this.

But for now, exercises that you can do easily from your house are things like:

Jogging on a spot

- ✓ Skipping
- ✓ Push ups
- ✓ Sit ups
- ✓ Taking walk.

EXERCISE REGULARLY.

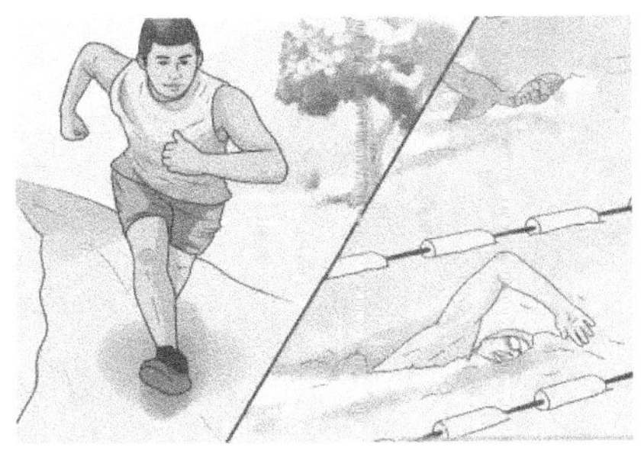

Moving your body enhances circulatory healthy, strengthening the arteries that carry blood to your penis. If you don't exercise at all, your penis may not be realizing its full potential. Aim to exercise for about an hour a day, whether you want to go for a swim, a walk, a jog or a bike ride. Any type of exercise will help increase blood flow to your penis.

- However, there's no way to exercise your penis itself in a way that will make it get bigger. The penis is composed of smooth muscle, which doesn't increase in mass with exercise.

Exercise Your Pelvic Floor.

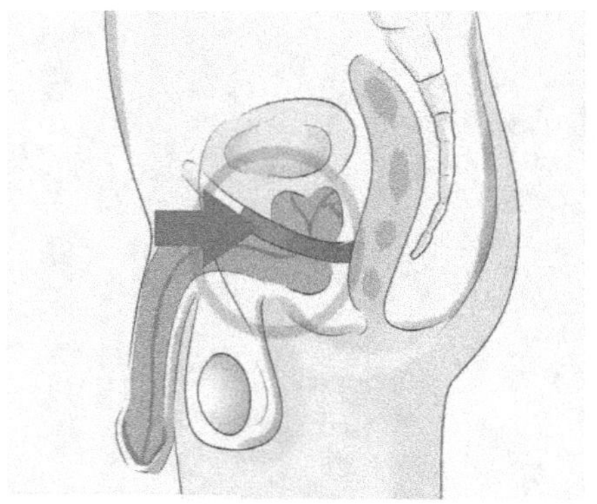

You may not be able to build up the penis itself through exercise, but if you strengthen your pelvic floor your body will be better able to hold blood in your penis. The pelvic floor presses on the vein that keeps blood from leaving the penis during erections. You can strengthen your pelvic floor using Kegel exercises. A trial conducted in Britain concluded that men who performed Kegel exercises experienced better sexual function than those who made other lifestyle changes but didn't perform the exercises.

- Find your pelvic floor by tightening the same muscle you use to stop your urine flow.
- Tighten and release the muscle 8 times. Rest and do it 8 more times, and again until you've done 3 or 4 sets.
- Do the exercises once a day for best results.

LOSE BELLY FAT & LOSING WEIGH

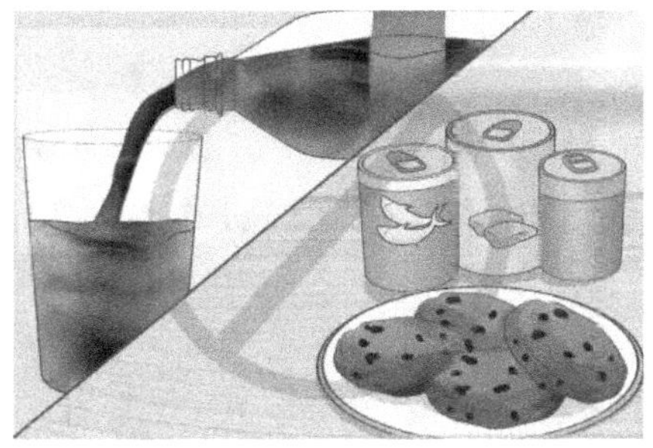

Your penis may look smaller than it really is if it's partially obscured by skin that droops over the top. Losing belly fat is no simple task, but it can make a big difference when it comes to the perceived size of your penis. Start taking measures to lose weight and you'll likely see improvement in other areas as well. According to a report from Harvard, men with a 42-inch waist are 50 percent more likely to have erectile dysfunction (ED) than men with a 32-inch waist.

- A regular exercise regimen will help you slim down. Aim to do cardio exercises as well as weight training.
- Eat whole foods, like lean meat, fish, whole grains, beans, legumes, vegetables, fruits and healthy oils.
- Avoid refined and processed foods, excessive sugar and starch, and hydrogenated oils.

For men who do have concerns about their penis size, doctors suggest that they start by losing weight. Although your penis won't actually get bigger, losing weight can reduce this pad of fat around the pubic bone, exposing more of the penis and making it appear larger . Even though it might not make your penis look longer, changes in your body can make it *look* that way.

You may even hear that losing 20-30 pounds will result in an extra inch of penis becoming visible or that being overweight hides up to 1/3 of your penis. While there no studies to back this up, it never hurts to lose weight and improving your health is good for your sex life, anyway!

LIPOSUCTION

As previously noted, gaining weight can result in the penis appearing shorter because the base becomes buried in fat. Liposuction may be used to reduce the pubic fat pad to make the penis appear larger. Studies show that suprapubic liposuction is very safe and successful with minor or no complications when it is performed meticulously, and long with improving associated esthetic concerns, it may help improve self-esteem as well

TRIMMING PUBIC HAIR

Pubic hair grooming in men has increased, with recent surveys finding that 50.5% of men surveyed reported regular pubic hair grooming. While men groom their pubic hair for many different reasons, from regular hygiene to making oral sex easier, improved appearance and making the penis look longer were found to be fairly common reasons for male grooming. Trimming pubic hair, particularly around the base of the penis, may give you the appearance of a larger penis.

PREVENTING SHRINKAGE

If you're worried about how to get a bigger penis, it's also a good idea to learn about issues that can cause penis shrinkage and learn how to prevent them. Certain medications, surgical procedures, and medical conditions have the ability to result in shrinkage. Here's a look at some of the potential causes of shrinkage and what you can do to prevent it.

PART 3

KNOWING WHAT TO AVOID

<u>Practises To Avoid</u>

There are different enlargement practises and methods worldwide in this world fastest growing industry. As a result many products has been introduced into the market with view of making some cool cash from unsuspecting insecure men. These are some practises you should avoid to keep safe.

STOP SMOKING-Beside the obvious health risks of smoking, studies show that smoking plays a major role in erectile & impotence problems among men.

And don't tell me about the nonsense that "Rolling Dollar (you know that old musician)" still smokes even in his 80s and is said to be strong sexually.

Well, a few people might be lucky but it doesn't mean you are one of those people.

So take proper precautions. It will help you on the long term.

Finally, the best piece of advice that can be given (and one you probably won't have any problem with) is this:

If you want to have better erections- <u>simple have MORE erections</u>!

The muscle tissue in your penis needs oxygen to survive. Where does it get that oxygen?

From the red blood cells flowing in the blood, the more blood that circulates, the less chance of erectile failure.

Since blood flows to the penis at a much greater rate when you have an erection, the best way to keep the muscle tissue in your penis properly oxygenated is by having more erections.

So, try to find a way to get more erections throughout the day and you will soon discover that you will begin to have better erections and this will keep you from having the same type of erection problems that most men suffer frcm.

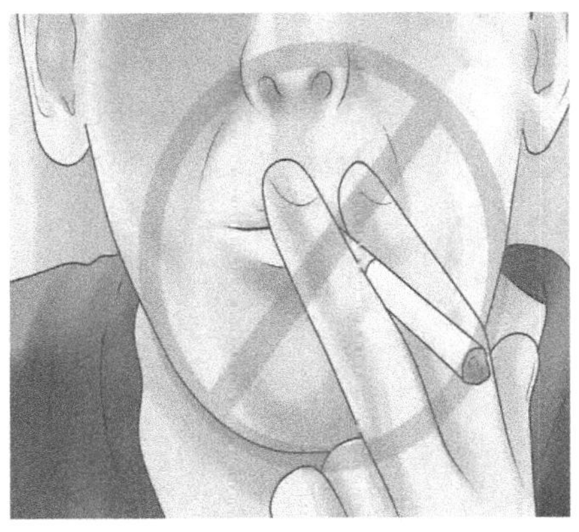

The size of your penis, whether it's flaccid or erect, depends on how much blood it contains. Using tobacco products causes the body's arteries to become narrower, which in turn reduces blood flow to the penis. If you smoke, you're inhibiting your penis from being as large as it could be.

VACUUM PUMPS

Try penis-enhancing devices.

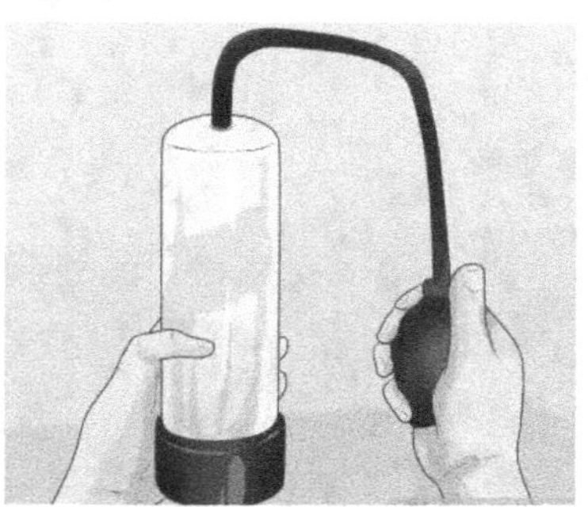

There are a few simple, non-invasive devices you can use to help your penis grow and stay enlarged long enough to have sex. If your aim is to have a bigger, firmer erection without using drugs or invasive treatments, try one of these devices:

- A penis ring. This works by holding blood in the penis when it becomes engorged during an erection. Your penis will temporarily be larger and stiffer.

- A penis pump. It's a vacuum device that fits around the penis. When you operate a hand pump, it draws blood into the penis and keeps it erect temporarily.

Vacuum pumps are often used to treat erectile dysfunction because they draw blood into the penis, causing it to swell. Some men have tried to use vacuum pumps to increase size, but routinely using a penis pump or using it longer than typically used to treat ED can result in damage to the elastic tissue of the penis, resulting in less-firm erections. Although a vacuum pump may create the illusion of a larger penis at the time, the results are not permanent.

Pumps have been made popular by adult stars who claim their large penises were a result of regular use of penis pumps. Notice, these adult stars almost always have impressively large penis to get into the profession. The only reason they use those pumps is to gain fullest extent erection long enough to perform their scene.

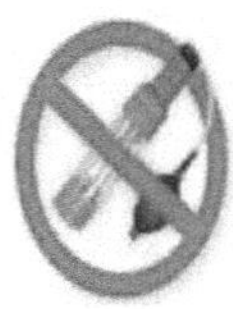 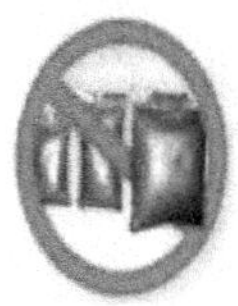

Pumps helps men with impotence since they force blood into the penis, which can result to a larger than normal, stronger erection. However the effects of pumps are temporary, they gain erection for minutes but do very little for long term penis enlargement.

Pumps causes series of negative side effects for men who choose to use them. For newbie, the mechanical forcing of blood into the penis is difficult to control often leaving him with severe bruises, blisters even bursts blood vessels within the penis region.

It is also called a "penis pump", a vacuum erection device, or VED, it creates negative pressure that expands and thereby draws blood into the penis. Medically approved VEDs, which treat erectile dysfunction, limit maximum pressure, whereas the pumps commonly bought by consumers seeking penis enlargement can reach dangerous pressure, damaging peris tissue. To retain tumescence after breaking the device's airtight seal, one must constrict the penis' base, but constriction worn over 30 minutes can permanently damage the penis and cause erectile dysfunction. Although vacuum therapy can treat erectile dysfunction sufficiently to prevent penis deterioration and shrinkage, clinical trials have not found it effective for penis enlargement.

Constant use may lead to impotence when the body begins to rely on mechanical stimulation to produce an erection, more includes deformation and diseases.

PILLS AND CREAMS: A lot of scams has come up in the media in the name of "magic pills" often with the claims of adding several inches, curing erectile dysfunction and quick ejaculation.

Reliable pills can work by increasing blood flow, which with the exercises results to quicker gains, the truth is that pills on their own cannot enlarge the penis, but can be used as supplement not a must use. Pills used in conjunction with the right penis enlargement exercises can speed up and enhance gains.

The internet is packed with banner ads and pop-ups that advertise pills and lotions for male enhancement and enlarging the penis. They often contain herbs, hormones, minerals, and vitamins, but none of them have been proven to work. Some pills have been investigated by the FDA and found to have levels of prescription drugs like sildenafil (Viagra) in them, and the FDA notes that there's a growing trend of dietary supplements that contain hidden chemicals and drugs.

With no proof to back them up and the potential dangers that come with hidden ingredients, we don't recommend these products if you want to grow your penis. There's no guarantee that they'll increase penis size, and you may experience unwanted side effects.

WEIGHTS: Weights can be dated a long time, probably the oldest penis enlargement technique, and the less complex to undergo.

Hanging weights has been found to be a dangerous technique for penis enlargement because of the amount of weight needed to gain a permanent effect.

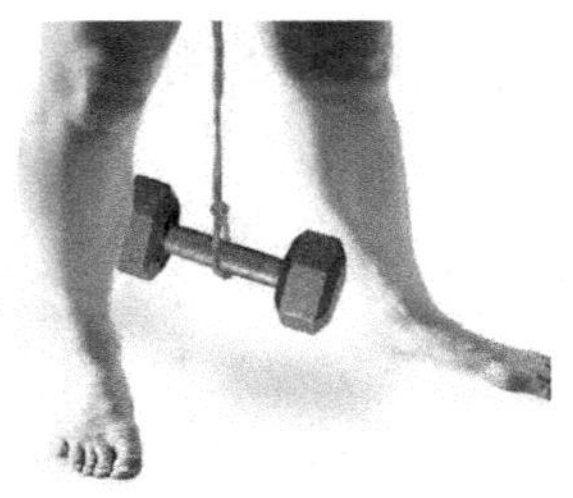

Research has the known dangers to include; painful erection, deformity and stretch marks, impotence, ligament damage and by stretching the penis in one direction any gains in length is most likely to be at the expense of girth which results to long thinner penis.

SURGERY: This is the most dangerous and the newest practise to emerge. Surgery, surgery is not only for the filthy rich, also not very safe and not under the control of the patient. The result of any plastic surgery is most times unpredictable and has increased chances of going wrong, plus possible futuristic complications.

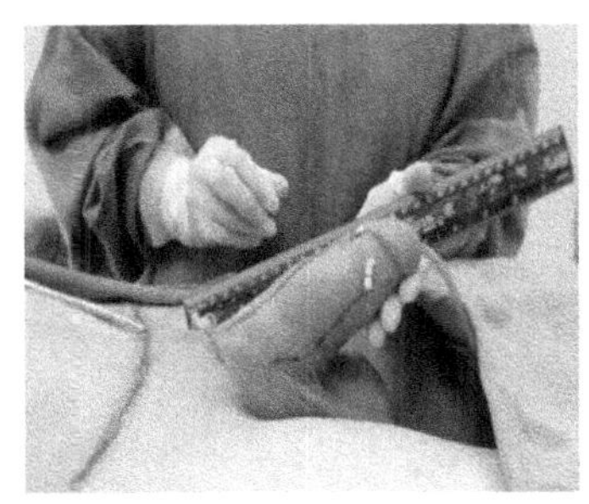

Surgery is an option for the rich who can afford the best surgeons around to enlarge their penises. Any mistake in the process could lead to impotence and put an end to your sex life. No surgeon can guarantee results, it's usually under probability.

Think it through carefully before getting surgery.

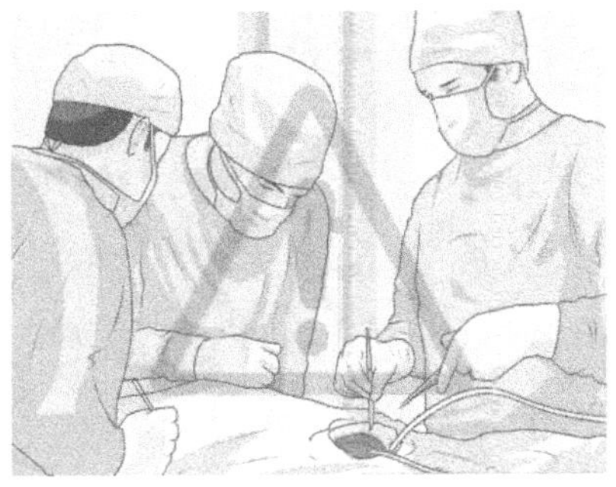

Surgical penis enlargement, or phalloplasty, has unfortunate side effects. The penis is extended in length, but you sacrifice function. After an enlargement procedure the penis is no longer able to stand out from the body; instead, it hangs between the legs. And sometimes, it no longer gets erect at all. Looking into natural solutions is a much better bet.

- Phalloplasty is used to build up a very small penis, also called a "micropenis," and in these cases the surgery is beneficial. However, phalloplasty performed on an average-length penis can lead to erectile dysfunction, scarring and deformity.

Which explains that even the surgeons carrying out the procedure do not have complete confidence in what they are doing, furthermore, surgery gone wrong is often irreversible; so it makes no sense taking this big risk.

So since we do not trust pills and creams, surgery and weight has such bad odds, then natural penis enlargement exercise using the hand is our best shot.

- You can perform at your leisure
- In your privacy and discretion
- You have total control of the process
- Whenever you feel like.

The truth is there is no miracle, magic or short cut to real penis enlargement.

I am delighted to show you how to make your own penis bigger, stronger and longer lasting. You will be proud and amazed at your manhood and confident of yourself than ever before.

There are two main types of penis enlargement surgery.

Penile augmentation involves injecting fat cells into the pen s. The aim is to increase girth, or width, as well as length, in some cases

The procedure carries risks. Side effects may include swelling and distortion of the penis. If a side effect is severe, the penis may require removal.

Another method of penile augmentation involves grafting fat cells from elsewhere in the body onto the penis. This is less invasive and can add an average of 2.39–2.65 cm after 12 months.

However, the organ can lose 20–80 percent of the new volume within 1 year of surgery, so people may need multiple surgeries to achieve the desired result.

The second main type of surgery is suspensory ligament release. This ligament anchors the penis to the pubic area and provides support during an erection. If a surgeon cuts the ligament, this changes the angle of the penis, which can make it look longer.

On average, suspensory ligament release can increase flaccid penis length by between 1–3 cm, but patient and partner satisfaction rates tend to be low. The lack of support during an erection can make penetration difficult.

Like the Urology Care Foundation, the American Urological Association states that penile augmentation surgery is neither safe nor effective.

STAY AWAY FROM PRODUCTS CLAIMING TO INCREASE PENIS SIZE.

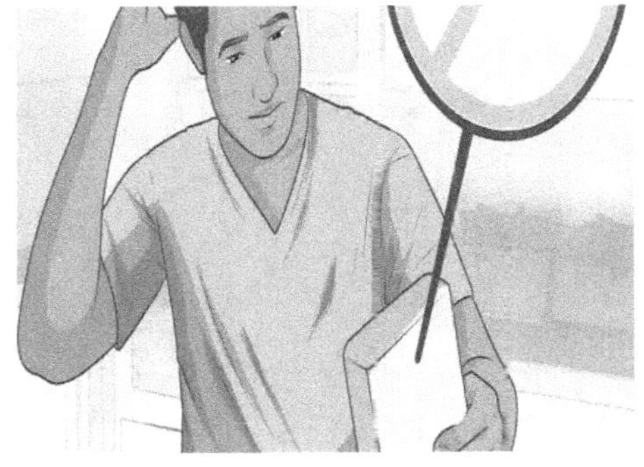

Since wanting a larger penis is such a common desire, there are a lot of scammers out there making promises they can't back up. There is no magic potion that will make your penis grow. It's completely genetic. Don't waste your money or jeopardize your health by falling prey to a company that promises to permanently give you a bigger penis with its product.

Be wary of "herbal Viagra" products.

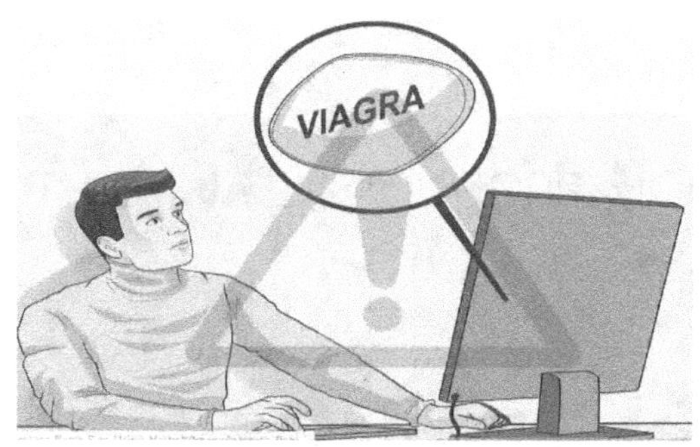

These are cocktails of the herbs known to increase blood flow to the penis, but since they aren't regulated by the FDA, it's difficult to know what the side effects might be. It's better to try herbs one at a time, controlling your dosage so that you don't accidentally take too much.

- Avoid ordering products online, even if the site selling them looks legitimate.
- If you do end up buying such a product, be cautious. Be sure not to try any type of penis-enhancement product until you check with your doctor.

Don't bother with stretching or weight-hanging.

These two techniques are said to lengthen the penis, and in some cases they do. But the longer it gets, the thinner it gets; both methods cause the penis to lose girth as it stretches out. The only time to use a penis stretcher is after having surgery, when it's necessary to prevent the accumulation of scar tissue.

This manual was created for informational purposes only and it is the responsibility of the user to thoroughly read the safety, warm-up, warm-down procedures prior to beginning this program.

As a result, the creator of this manual is not liable for any misuse or damage resulting from the contents in this manual.

The exercise techniques, if used improperly can damage the penis. This manual clearly indicates any possible safety issues that may arise while using this product.

The creator of this guide is not a certified medical practitioner.

So, make sure you consult a professional medical practitioner for professional advice before you start to apply any of the instructions contained in this manual.

GOODLUCK!!!